A KNOWLEDGE, ATTITUDE & PRACTICES (KAP) SURVEY OF BIOMEDICAL WASTE DISPOSAL IN HAYATABAD MEDICAL COMPLEX

PATRON:
PROFESSOR DR. BUSHRA IFTIKHAR
Head, Department of Community Medicine
Khyber Medical College, Peshawar.

SUPERVISOR:
PROFESSOR DR. BUSHRA IFTIKHAR
Head, Department of Community Medicine

SUBMITTED BY:
Batch 07 (Session 2013 - 2014)

DEPARTMENT OF COMMUNITY MEDICINE AND PUBLIC HEALTH
KHYBER MEDICAL COLLEGE
PESHAWAR

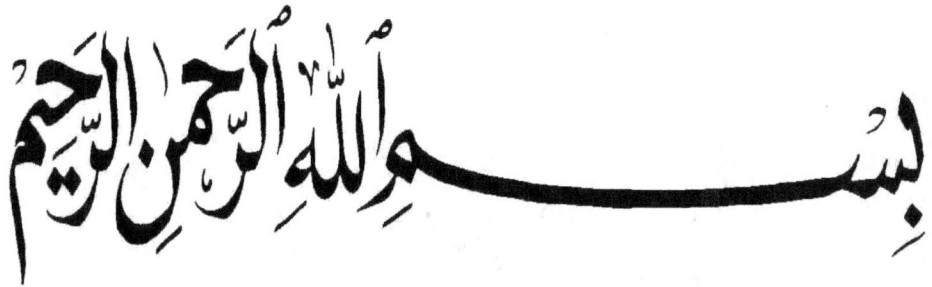

In the Name of Allah, the Most Gracious, the Most Merciful.

**AKNOWLEDGE, ATTITUDE & PRACTICES (KAP)
SURVEY OF BIOMEDICAL WASTE DISPOSAL IN HAYATABAD MEDICAL
COMPLEX**

CONTRIBUTIONS

**THE PROJECT WAS A SUCCESS BECAUSE OF THE DEDICATED
CONTRIBUTION AND HARD WORK OF THE FOLLOWING TEAM
MEMBERS:**

BATCH 7

**DEPARTMENT OF COMMUNITY MEDICINE
KHYBER MEDICAL COLLEGE PESHAWAR**

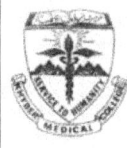

APPROVAL SHEET

It is stated that Batch No. 7 of 4th year MBBS of the session 2013-2014 of Khyber Medical College Peshawar is hereby given approval by the Department of Community Medicine, Khyber Medical College, Peshawar to do research work on the topic entitled "A Knowledge, Attitude & Practices (KAP) Survey of Biomedical Waste Disposal In Hayatabad Medical Complex" under the supervision of same department.

Patron in Chief   Project Supervisor

--------------------------------   --------------------------------

Professor Dr. Bushra Iftikhar   **Professor Dr. Bushra Iftikhar**
Head, Department of Community Medicine   Head Department of Community Medicine
Khyber Medical College, Peshawar   Khyber Medical College, Peshawar

DEPARTMENT OF COMMUNITY MEDICINE
KHYBER MEDICAL COLLEGE PESHAWAR

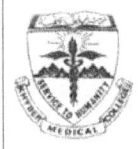

SUPERVISOR'S CERTIFICATE

This is to certify that the project entitled "A Knowledge, Attitude & Practices (KAP) Survey of Biomedical Waste Disposal in Hayatabad Medical Complex" is a bonafide record of research work done by Batch No. 7, 4th Year MBBS under my supervision during the session 2013-2014 submitted to the Department of Community Medicine.

I have thoroughly gone through the project work and found it very well.

Professor Dr. Bushra Iftikhar
Project Supervisor
Department of Community Medicine
Khyber Medical College, Peshawar.

ACKNOWLEDGEMENT

All the praises and thanks to Allah Almighty who enabled to carry out this project without any complications and in time.

This project would not have been possible without the help and support of a number of people. It is our privilege to express our heartfelt gratitude to our Head of Department, Dr. Bushra Iftikhar for enabling us to avail this golden opportunity to prepare a project and help us gain an experience that will brighten up and open up ways for our future of research.

Last, but not the least, we are truly grateful for the help provided by the staff of the wards of HMC. They helped us in every way possible in filling us in with the details of patients from whom the data was collected, without which this project would have been incomplete.

OBJECTIVES

1. To assess and evaluate the knowledge of the hospital staff regarding the biomedical waste disposal

2. To estimate the attitude of the staff regarding waste disposal

3. To compare the attitudes of Doctors, Nurses, Laboratory Technicians and Sanitary staff regarding waste disposal and management

4. The procedures and techniques which are adopted for the segregation, storage arrangements, collection and waste disposal

INTRODUCTION

Production of waste products is one of the chief characteristics of the living beings. All the living things produce waste products in some form or the other. This waste may be biodegradable or non-biodegradable. Normally, aerobic and anaerobic processes in the ecosystem degrade such products. However, the main threat to the environment is because of the non-biodegradable products which resist degradation by ordinary methods.

Biomedical waste which is also referred to as infectious waste or medical waste is defined as *"any waste which is generated in the diagnosis, treatment and immunization of human beings and animals in research pertaining thereto or in the production or testing of biological" (Standard Operating Procedures for Hospital Waste Management Government of Pakistan, 1996)[1]*. This biomedical waste is not an ordinary waste but it is a waste of special and unique importance by virtue of its source of production, composition, its hazard which needs special precautions while handling, its disposal which requires multistep techniques and scientific procedures and the threats it poses to the public health and environment, if this waste is not disposed of properly. Improper handling and mismanagement during the treatment and disposal of this waste not only put at risk the life of the staff handling it but also the general public and the environment as well.

Hospital is a place to serve the patient and address his/her health problems and exercise all those means and ways to provide ailment and relief his suffering.

In the beginning, the hospitals were known just for the treatment of sick persons and didn't have the complex functional and operational structure and therefore, we were unaware about the adverse effects of the waste generated by them and its ultimate impact on human body and environment. Now it is a well-established and a proven fact that there are many adverse and harmful effects to the environment including human beings which are caused by the "Biomedical waste" generated during the delivery of health care to the patients. Hospital waste is a potential health hazard to the health care workers, the waste management staff, public, flora and fauna of the area and to the environment. Hospital acquired infections, transfusion transmitted diseases, rising incidence of Hepatitis B, and HIV, increasing land and water pollution lead to increasing possibility of catching many diseases. Air pollution due to emission of hazardous gases by incinerator such as Furan, Dioxin, Hydrochloric acid etc. have compelled the authorities to think seriously about hospital waste and the diseases transmitted through improper disposal of hospital waste[2]. This problem has now become a serious threat for the public.

A modern hospital is a complex, multidisciplinary system which consumes thousands of items for delivery of medical care and is a part of physical environment. All these products consumed in the hospital leave some unusable leftovers i.e. hospital waste. In the last century a rapid growth of hospital in the public and private sector occurred, so as to provide preventive, diagnostic and treatment facilities to the rapidly growing population and cope with the modern day challenges and disease burden of communicable and non-communicable diseases. The advent and acceptance of "disposable" has made the generation of hospital waste a significant factor in current scenario and greatly increased the amount of waste of hospitals.

The biomedical waste is a burning issue of modern era because of its relation to health and environment. Efforts are made to reduce the quantity of the waste produced. The principle of reuse and recycle is taking popularity.

CLASSIFICATION OF HOSPITAL WASTE

Hospital waste refers to all waste generated in the hospital that is of no further use, needs to be discarded and disposed and it can be classified as

(1)   **General waste:** Largely composed of domestic or house hold type waste. It is non-hazardous to human beings, e.g. kitchen waste, packaging material, paper, wrappers, and plastics.

(2)   **Pathological waste:** Consists of tissue, organ, body part, human foetuses, blood and body fluid. It is hazardous waste.

(3)   **Infectious waste:** The wastes which contain pathogens in sufficient concentration or quantity that could cause diseases. It is hazardous e.g. culture and stocks of infectious agents from laboratories, waste from surgery, waste originating from infectious patients.

(4)   **Sharps:** Waste materials which could cause the person handling it, a cut or puncture of skin e.g. needles, broken glass, saws, nail, blades, and scalpels.

(5)   **Pharmaceutical waste:** This includes pharmaceutical products, drugs, and chemicals that have been returned from wards, have been spilled, are out-dated, or contaminated.

(6)   **Chemical waste:** This comprises discarded solid, liquid and gaseous chemicals e.g. cleaning, housekeeping, and disinfecting product.

(7)   **Radioactive waste:** It includes solid, liquid, and gaseous waste that is contaminated with radionuclides generated from in-vitro analysis of body tissues and fluid, in-vivo body organ imaging and tumour localization and therapeutic procedures.

(8)   **Pressurized containers:** Containers containing a liquid or gas under pressure[2].

Rationale of hospital waste management

Hospital waste management is a part of hospital hygiene and maintenance activities and is of prime importance in order to enable the delivery of health care smoothly and safely. In fact only 15% of hospital waste i.e. "Biomedical waste" is hazardous, not the complete[2]. But when hazardous waste is not segregated at the source of generation and mixed with non-hazardous waste, then 100% waste becomes hazardous. Spending so many resources in terms of money, man power, material and machine for management of hospital waste? The reasons are:

·   Injuries from sharps leading to infection to all categories of hospital personnel and waste handler.

·   Nosocomial infections in patients from poor infection control practices and poor waste management.

·   Risk of infection outside hospital for waste handlers and scavengers and at time general public living in the vicinity of hospitals.

·   Risk associated with hazardous chemicals, drugs to persons handling wastes at all levels.

·   Disposable items being repacked and sold by unscrupulous elements without even being washed.

·   Drugs which have been disposed of, being repacked and sold off to unsuspecting buyers.

·   Risk of air, water and soil pollution directly due to waste, or due to defective incineration emissions and ash.

Problems relating to biomedical waste

A major issue related to current Bio-Medical waste management in many hospitals is that the implementation of Bio-Waste regulation is unsatisfactory as some hospitals are disposing of waste in a haphazard, improper and indiscriminate manner. Lack of segregation practices, results in mixing of hospital wastes with general waste making the whole waste stream hazardous. Inappropriate segregation ultimately results in an incorrect method of waste disposal.

Inadequate Bio-Medical waste management thus will cause environmental pollution, unpleasant smell, growth and multiplication of vectors like insects, rodents and worms and may lead to the transmission of diseases like typhoid, cholera, hepatitis and AIDS through injuries from syringes and needles contaminated with human[3].

Various communicable diseases, which spread through water, sweat, blood, body fluids and contaminated organs, are important to be prevented. The Bio Medical Waste scattered in and around the hospitals invites flies, insects, rodents, cats and dogs that are responsible for the spread of communication disease like plague and rabies. Rag pickers in the hospital, sorting out the garbage are at a risk of getting tetanus and HIV infections. The recycling of disposable syringes, needles, IV sets and other article like glass bottles without proper sterilization are responsible for Hepatitis, HIV, and other viral diseases. It becomes primary responsibility of Health administrators to manage hospital waste in most safe and eco-friendly manner[3].

The problem of bio-medical waste disposal in the hospitals and other healthcare establishments has become an issue of increasing concern, prompting hospital administration to seek new ways of scientific, safe and cost effective management of the waste, and keeping their personnel informed about the advances in this area. The need of proper hospital waste management system is of prime importance and is an essential component of quality assurance in hospitals.

METHODOLOGY

Study Design

This was a direct observational cross sectional study aiming at the assessment of

the knowledge and attitude of hospital staff regarding biomedical waste

management and disposal and the prevailing health care waste handling,

management and treatment system in a tertiary care hospital of Peshawar, the

Hayatabad Medical Complex

Study Area

Hayatabad Medical Complex is a teaching hospital offering primary, tertiary, and

quaternary care not only to the citizens of Khyber Pakhtunkhwa but also to those

of the adjoining tribal areas of FATA and Afghanistan. The hospital caters for a

population of approximately 30 million people. Located in Phase-4 Hayatabad,

HMC covers an area total of 351 Kanals of land (215 Kanals was acquired in 1985

and 136 Kanals in 1987).Decision to convert it into a general hospital was taken in

1993 and its 1st Phase was inaugurated with 289 beds in August 1996. The hospital

was operational in February 1997 HMC have a total Staff of 1215, consisting of

200 Doctors and 190 TMOs , 401 nursing staff, 194 Paramedical staff,53

ministerial/accounts staff, 26 technical staff and 341 auxiliary staff. The hospital

comprises of a 720 beds hospital, clinical units of Post Graduate Medical Institute

(PGMI), Institute of Kidney Diseases (IKD), Pakistan Institute of Community

Ophthalmology (PICO) and Khyber Girls Medical College (KGMC).Hayatabad Medical Complex offers a full range of emergency and high dependency care in Maternity, Pediatrics, Surgery, Orthopedics and Medicine. Sub specialty care like Endocrinology, Ophthalmology, ENT, Pediatric cardiology, Cardiology, Gastroenterology, Plastic Surgery and Neurosurgery are services are also provided. The hospital also has a Radiology department where X-ray and CT-Scan services are available, a pathology department and a Physiotherapy Unit. With the vision "To be the model of excellence for health services delivery, meeting the needs and enhancing the health of the people of KPK" HMC takes part in numerous vertical programs like HIV/AIDS control programme, Reproductive Family health centre, Prevention of parent to child transmission center, Prime Minister's programme for control and prevention of Hepatitis ,National TB control programme, Expanded programme on Immunization (EPI) , and is working on developing sophisticated and new resources such as a Level I Trauma Center, Regional Burn Center, and a BSL-3 regional TB laboratory etc, proving its excellence in level of care the hospital offers to inpatients as well as outpatients through its extensive clinic system[14].

Study Population

The study population consisted of doctors, nurses, laboratory technicians and sanitary staff (sweepers).

Sample Size

Data was collected from a sample size of 200. It consisted of 60 doctors, 60 nurses, 40 laboratory technicians and 40 sanitary staff (sweepers).

Sampling Technique

The population is 1215 staff members of Hayatabad Medical Complex Peshawar, out of which 200 are doctors, 190 TMOs, 400 nurses, 194 paramedical staff, 48 ministerial staff, 05 finance/account staff, 26 technical staff and 365 auxiliary staff.

The sample size selected is 200 out of 1215 staff members, which will include 60 doctors, 60 nurses, 40 lab technicians and 40 sanitation staff.

For The selection of Doctors and Nurses Multistage Sampling Design was adopted.

First Stage Sampling includes Selection of wards. We had received the list of all the wards/units of the Institute From hospital administration and out which 12 such units were selected by simple random sampling which includes 2 medical ,2 surgical ,2 gynaecology ,1 nephrology, 1 orthopedic,1 cardiology,1 urology, 1 ENT and 1 Gastroenterology ward.

Second stage sampling includes selection of doctors and nurses. A list of doctors and nurses of all in-patients units (mentioned above) of the Institute were enumerated was obtained from the hospital administration.5 doctors and 5 nurses were selected by Simple random sampling from each of the 12 selected units.

For the selection of Lab technicians and sanitation staff, simple random sampling design was adopted. A list of all the lab technicians (working in Chemical Pathology, Haematology, Microbiology and Histopathology) and sanitation staff was obtained from the Institute Administration. Total of 40 lab technicians out of 50 and 40 sanitation staff out of 135 were selected by simple random selection.

Data Collection:

Data regarding this study was collected through a structured questionnaire which consisted of both open and closed ended and questions and an observation checklist.

The questionnaire was divided into three sections i.e. knowledge, attitude and practices section. The knowledge section comprised of 10 questions regarding the knowledge about biomedical waste. In the attitude section, a structured five-point Likert Scale questionnaire was used as the study tool. The scores were from +5 for the most positive response to +1 for the least positive. There were seven questions related to the measurement of attitude. The score on the scale is the ratings for each item and finally the sum of the scores of all the items ("summated" scale). The items that are reversed in meaning from the overall direction of the scale are reversal items. The response value is reversed for each of these items. The minimum and maximum possible summated attitude scores were +7 and +35. The practices section comprised of 2 questions questionnaire was formatted in a simple fashion to make it easier while answering the questions.

An observational checklist was designed and used to evaluate the methods practiced for the collection, segregation, packaging, storage arrangements treatment and waste disposal.

a. Personal visits to the hospital were made and doctors, nurses, laboratory technicians and sanitary staff (sweepers) were personally interviewed.

b. Personal observations were made and information given in the questionnaire was counter checked.

c. A personal visit to the waste treatment site was made to see the ultimate disposal of health care waste over there.

Data Analysis

SPSS and Microsoft Excel were used for the analysis of data.

Work Plan

The research was completed in the time frame of February 2013 to September 2013. The topic was selected in the month of February. Questionnaire was designed in March. From April to July the introduction was completed. Data was collected in the last week of August and in first week of September. The results, analysis, discussion, conclusion and literature review was completed in the 2nd week of September. After that it was given for printing.

Financing

The project was self-funded. Fund was raised by mutual contribution of all batch members to meet the expenses.

LITERATURE REVIEW

Medical care is an essential need and requirement for our life and health, but it is the waste generated during the delivery of health care which creates a problem for us and require our attention for its safe handling, management and disposal. Improper management of waste generated in health care facilities causes a direct health impact on the community, the health care workers and on the environment. Relatively large amount of potentially infectious and hazardous waste are generated in the health care hospitals and facilities around the world on daily basis. Indiscriminate and improper disposal this biomedical or hospital waste and exposure to such waste possess serious threat to environment and to human health that requires specific treatment and management prior to its final disposal. Healthcare waste is defined as the total waste stream from a healthcare facility. There are two basic categories of this waste

- Healthcare General Waste

- Healthcare Risk Waste

- Healthcare General Waste include

  - Paper Packaging

  - Plastic packaging

  - Food preparation

- And other items that haven't been contaminated

- Healthcare Risk Waste include

    - Infectious waste

    - Hazardous waste

    - Harmful to humans and environment

Sources of Biomedical Waste

Hospitals produce waste, which is increasing over the years in its amount and type. The hospital waste, in addition to the risk for patients and personnel who handle them, also poses a threat to public health and environment.

Major Sources

- Govt. hospitals/private hospitals/nursing homes/ dispensaries.
- Primary health centres.
- Medical colleges and research centres/ paramedic services.
- Veterinary colleges and animal research centres.
- Blood banks/mortuaries/autopsy centres.
- Biotechnology institutions.
- Production units.

Minor Sources

- Physicians/ dentists' clinics

- Animal houses/slaughter houses.

- Blood donation camps.

- Vaccination centres.

- Acupuncturists/psychiatric clinics/cosmetic piercing.

- Funeral services.

- Institutions for disabled persons[3]

Amount and composition of hospital waste generated
(a) Amount

Country	Quantity (kg/bed/day)
U. K[2].	2.5
U.S.A[2].	4.5
France[2]	2.5
Spain[2]	3.0
India[2]	1.5
Pakistan[4]	2.0

(b) Composition

Of this 2.0kg/bed/day hospital waste generated 0.1-0.5 can be categorized as risk waste[4].

In 2001, during measles mass immunization campaign in West Africa (covering all or part of six countries), 17 million children were vaccinated, resulting in the generation of nearly 300 metric tonnes of injection waste. Without adequate waste disposal options at both local and regional levels, this volume of waste would have been difficult to eliminate safely[5].

The unsafe disposal of health-care waste (for example, contaminated syringes and needles) poses public health risks and also affects the flora, fauna and environment. Contaminated needles and syringes represent a particular threat as the failure to dispose of them safely may lead to dangerous recycling and repackaging which lead to unsafe reuse. Contaminated injection equipment may be scavenged from waste areas and dumpsites and either be reused or sold to be used again. WHO estimated that, in 2000, contaminated injections with contaminated syringes caused:

- 21 million hepatitis B virus (HBV) infections (32% of all new infections);
- two million hepatitis C virus (HCV) infections (40% of all new infections); and
- at least 260 000 HIV infections (5% of all new infections)[12].

In 2002, the results of a WHO assessment conducted in 22 developing countries showed that the proportion of health-care facilities that do not use proper waste disposal methods ranges from 18% to 64%[5].

In addition to the public health risks, if not managed, direct reuse of contaminated injection equipment results in occupational hazards to health workers, waste handlers and scavengers. Where waste is dumped into areas without restricted access, children may come into contact with contaminated waste and play with used needles and syringes. Epidemiological studies indicate that a person who experiences one needle stick injury from a needle used on an infected source patient has risks of 30%, 1.8%, and 0.3% respectively of becoming infected with HBV, HCV and HIV[5].

There are Guidelines for Hospital Waste Management in Pakistan since 1998 prepared by the Environmental Health Unit, of the Ministry of Health, Government of Pakistan, giving detailed information and covering all aspects of safe hospital waste management in the country, including the risk associated with the waste, formation of a waste management team in hospitals, their responsibilities, plan, collection, segregation, transportation, storage, disposal methods, containers, and their color-coding, waste minimization techniques, protective clothing, etc. It is unfortunate that many hospitals and cities in Pakistan are facing serious problems. There are no systematic approaches to medical waste disposal. Hospital wastes are simply mixed with the municipal waste in collecting bins at roadsides and disposed of similarly. Some waste is simply buried without any appropriate measure. In Pakistan, despite the existence of Pakistan Biosafety Rules 2005 (SRO 2005) neither proper hospital waste management system have been developed in various health institutions nor the concerned health professionals are aware of the situation resulting. So the disposal of hospital waste is a serious problem in Pakistan[6]. Every hospital shall be responsible for the proper management of the waste generated by it till its final disposal[007]. Pakistan is in a phase of creating awareness and implementing hospital waste management techniques. The concerted efforts needed might fall short, if the attitudes of the staff and the public towards this, is not changed. In Pakistan usually two methods are being used to dispose off the hospital waste i.e. landfills and incineration. In landfill method, hospital waste is buried underground but according to health experts not a single landfill is constructed on scientific lines. Incinerators installed at various places also do not have proper filters and scrubbers and when hospital waste is burnt, toxic gases like dioxin and chemicals are discharged in the air which can be potential carcinogen. Only a few hospitals have proper incinerators. Health experts recommend that the hospital waste should be segregated from the solid waste and stored in special containers. Proper landfills should be constructed and all incinerators working without filters and scrubbers should be immediately shut down.

The National Program for Prevention Control of Hepatitis is in the process of developing national guidelines. The program has also developed Trainer's and Trainees Manuals for various categories of healthcare workers including health managers, professionals and the auxiliary as well as waste management staff.

National guidelines have been developed for hospital waste management where great emphasis is laid on minimizing waste generation, segregation, storage before disposal, appropriate disposal methods for various waste categories and above all supervision, monitoring & evaluation of the entire process. The training is also being made mandatory focusing on health managers, medical professionals, paramedics and waste management staff.

Planning Commission had envisioned the severity of the problem and addressed the issues related to hospital waste in its next 5 years plan (2005-10) through capacity building, finalization of rules on hazardous waste, creating inventory of hazardous waste. Similarly funding is allocated for management of hospital waste in various projects pertaining to different hospitals and projects executers.

Since the overall goal of waste management is to prevent disease transmission from waste products, therefore, emphasis should be placed more on the "Management" aspect of the process and not on the "technological" aspect which is expensive diversion rather than an effective solution. Technology must be compatible with the situation and should work in the management system to achieve the desired goal as a part of overall system and not as a replacement alternate. Technology choices must be according to local needs and conditions and its affordability in sustained manner. Therefore, based on the information presented in this is paper, it is recommended that a "Hospital Waste Management System in Pakistan" should be established with the following considerations:

·   Comprehensive analysis of the current hospital waste management practices in public and private sectors.

·   National policy for establishment of hospital waste management system in Pakistan.

·   Include hospital based management as priority area in Medium Term Development Framework 2010-15 with a clear plan of action for implementation.

·   Design mega development project for safe disposal and management of hospital waste.

·   Identification of National Core Group who can provide guidance in establishing hospital waste management system in the country.

·   Development of strategic framework involving all stakeholders (public and private sectors as well as international agencies).

·   Advocacy, awareness and training of hospital professionals and other staff about proper hospital waste disposal.

· Implementation of hospital waste management guidelines developed by the Environment Protection Agency in 2005.

· Execution of National Hospital Waste Management Plan in line with the National Policy and the Strategic Framework.

· Monitoring and Evaluation of the Hospital Waste Management interventions.

Biomedical Waste Management Process

The hospital waste like body parts, organs, tissues, blood and body fluids along with soiled linen, cotton, bandage and plaster casts from infected and contaminated areas are very essential to be properly collected, segregated, stored, transported, treated and disposed of in safe manner to prevent nosocomial or hospital acquired infection and pollution of the environment.

1. Waste collection

2. Segregation at the source of production

3. Packaging and color-coding (labelling)

4. Transportation and storage

5. Treatment & Disposal

6. Transport to final disposal site

7. Final disposal

RESULTS

Demographics:

The demographic details of the sample are as under.

Gender Based Distribution of Sample

Sex	Position				Total
	Sanitary Staff	Lab Technician	Nurse	Doctor	
Male	100.0%	95.0%	0.0%	75.0%	61.5%
Female	0.0%	5.0%	100.0%	25.0%	38.5%

Education Based Distribution of Sample

Position	Education				
	Primary	Matric	HSSC	Graduation	Post-Graduation
Sanitary Staff	63.2%	26.3%	10.5%	0.0%	0.0%
Lab Technician	0.0%	5.0%	15.0%	70.0%	10.0%
Nurse	0.0%	3.3%	20.0%	68.3%	8.3%
Doctor	0.0%	0.0%	0.0%	51.7%	48.3%
Total	12.1%	7.1%	11.1%	50.5%	19.2%

Age Based Distribution

Age(in years)	Frequency	Percent	Valid Percent	Cumulative Percent
12 - 21	14	7.0	7.0	7.0
22 - 31	114	57.0	57.0	64.0
32 - 41	52	26.0	26.0	90.0
42 - 51	17	8.5	8.5	98.5
52+	3	1.5	1.5	100.0
Total	200	100.0	100.0	

Knowledge:

Position	Percentage who knew about biomedical waste
Sanitary Staff	5.0%
Lab Technician	70.0%
Nurse	8.3%
Doctor	91.7%

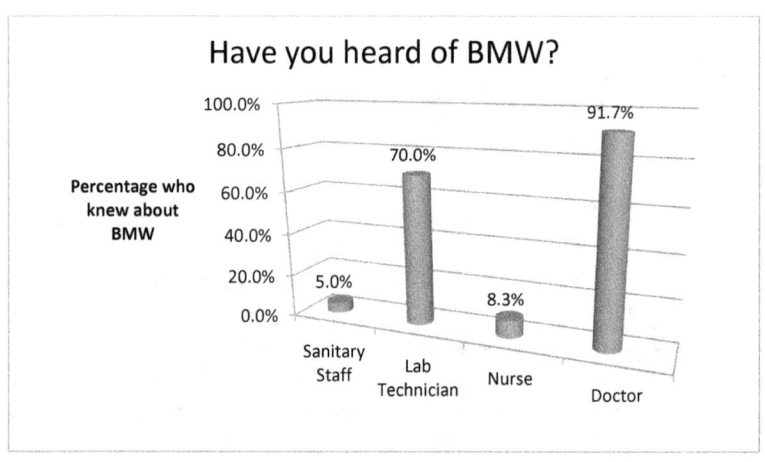

Position	Percentage who knew the biohazard symbol
Sanitary Staff	5.0%
Lab Technician	35.0%
Nurse	1.7%
Doctor	46.7%

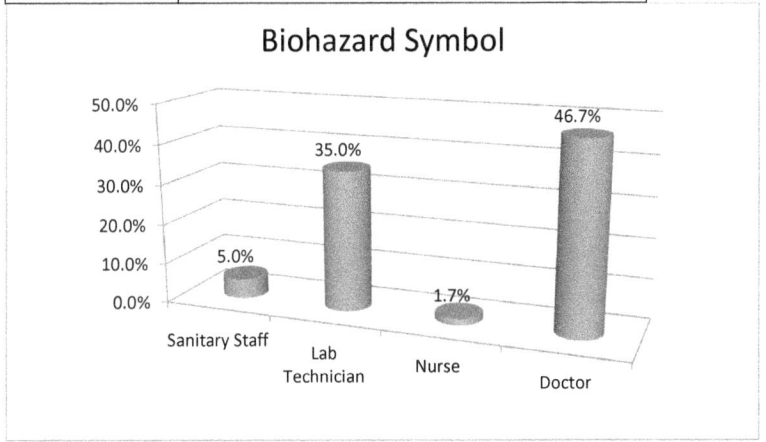

Position	Percentage aware of the fact improper management of waste causes different health problems
Sanitary Staff	90.0%
Lab Technician	100.0%
Nurse	100.0%
Doctor	96.7%

Percentage aware of the fact improper management of waste causes different health problems

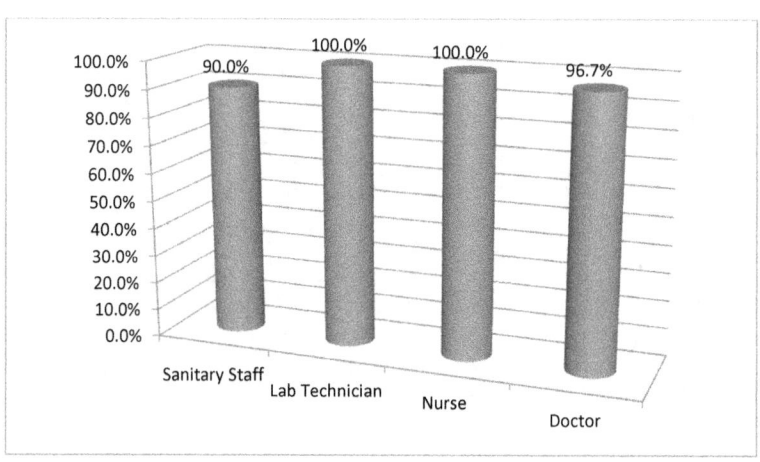

Position	Improper waste management may result in the disease			
	HIV	Hepatitis	Both HIV & Hepatitis	Other blood borne disease
Sanitary Staff	5.6%	5.6%	83.3%	5.6%
Lab Tech	10.5%	21.1%	68.4%	0.0%
Nurse	0.0%	3.3%	91.7%	5.0%
Doctor	0.0%	21.7%	75.0%	3.3%

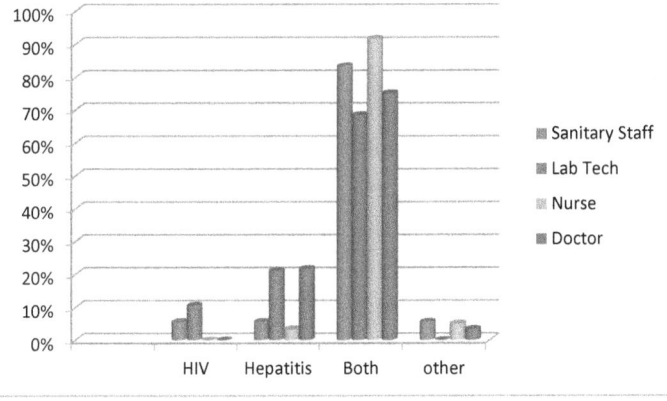

Position	Percentage knowing the use of color-coded bags for waste disposal
Sanitary Staff	2.5%
Lab Technician	10.0%
Nurse	1.7%
Doctor	25.0%

Position	Percentage who thinks there hospital has no waste management plan
Sanitary Staff	42.1%
Lab Technician	50.0%
Nurse	48.3%
Doctor	53.3%

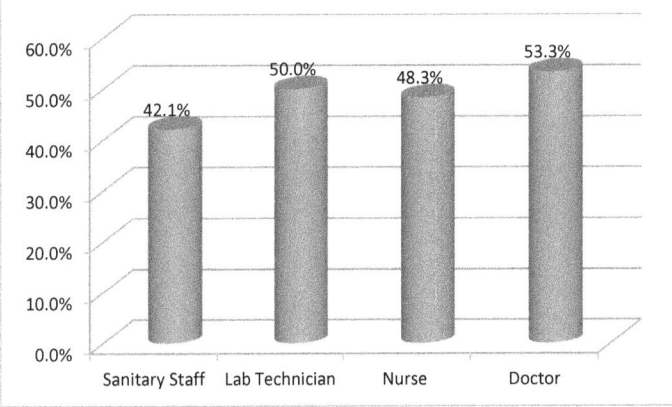

Are there clearly defined procedures for collection and handling of wastes from specified units in the hospital	
Position	Yes
Sanitary Staff	40.0%
Lab Technician	40.0%
Nurse	50.0%
Doctor	28.8%

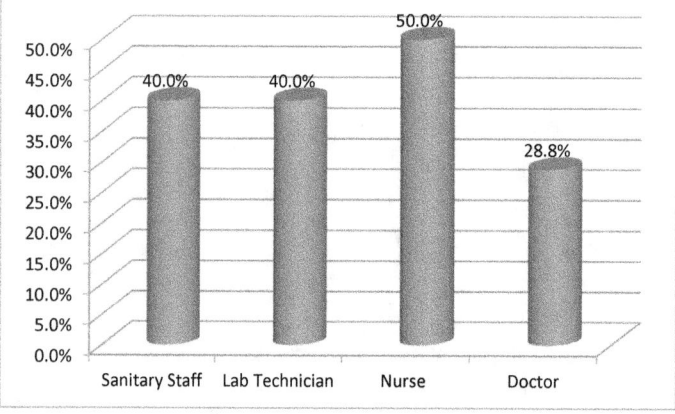

Position	Percentage who have received training/ attended workshop on waste handling and management
Sanitary Staff	10.0%
Lab Technician	15.0%
Nurse	21.7%
Doctor	11.7%

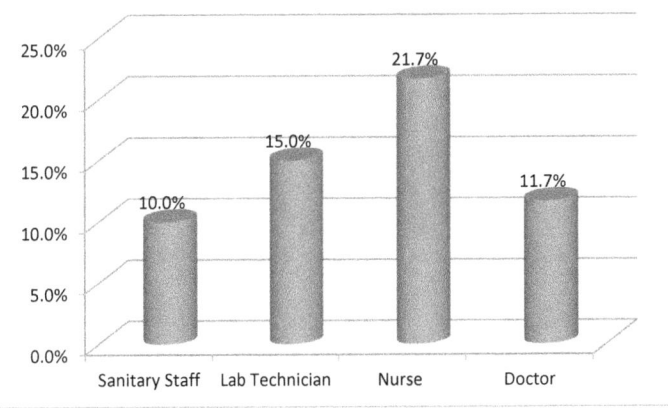

Are instructions/training given to newly hired waste management staff	
Yes	No
15.0%	85.0%

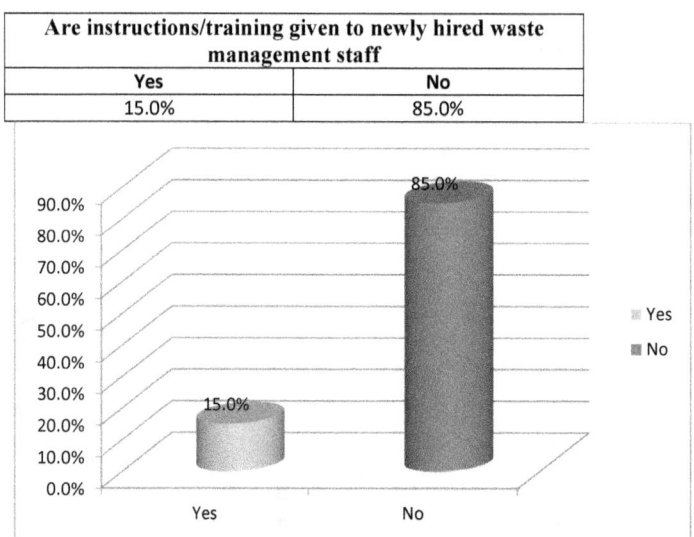

Attitude:

A structured five-point Likert Scale questionnaire was used as the study tool. The

scores were from +5 for the most positive response to +1 for the least positive.

There were seven questions related to the measurement of attitude. The score on

the scale is the ratings for each item and finally the sum of the scores of all the

items ("summated" scale). The items that are reversed in meaning from the

overall direction of the scale are reversal items. The response value is reversed for

each of these items. The minimum and maximum possible summated attitude

scores were +7 and +35.

The mean responses to the seven likert questions were summed for each

group and the summated attitude was obtained. The summated attitude scores of

the sanitary staff, lab technicians, nurses and doctors were 26.18, 28.65, 26.50

and 29.25 respectively as shown in the tables.

Statement	Position			
	Sanitary Staff	Lab Technician	Nurse	Doctor
Safe management of health care waste is an important issue	4.15	4.85	4.87	4.78
Management of healthcare waste is not the responsibility of Doctors/nurses/paramedic staff	3.23	3.65	3.48	3.82
Waste management is possible even in overcrowded hospitals of Peshawar	3.65	4.10	3.70	4.12
Waste management efforts by hospitals need unnecessary expenditure	3.68	3.85	3.67	3.83
Safe management of waste is an extra burden on over-worked hospital staff	3.60	3.35	2.40	4.05
Waste management is possible even when patients are poor and illiterate	3.88	4.10	3.48	4.13
Proper segregation and then properly managed and disposed waste decrease the likelihood of the disease risk from the waste	4.00	4.75	4.90	4.52
Summated Attitude	**26.18**	**28.65**	**26.50**	**29.25**

Summated Attitude			
Position	Mean	N	Std. Deviation
Sanitary Staff	26.18	40	2.01
Lab Technician	28.65	40	2.44
Nurse	26.50	60	3.44
Doctor	29.25	60	3.44
Overall	27.69	200	3.28

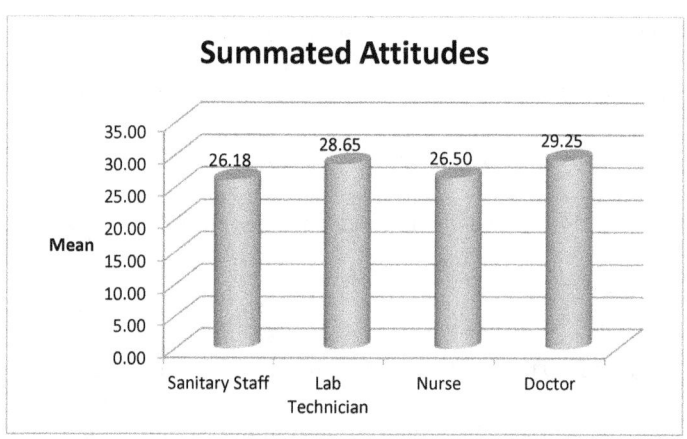

A one way ANOVA test of these summated attitudes showed that the differences between attitude of different groups (Sanitary Staff, Laboratory Technicians, Nurses, Doctors) is statistically significant ($P < 0.05$). The difference between the overall (mean) summated attitude score (27.69) and the maximum possible summated attitude score (35) is also statistically significant ($P < 0.05$).

There was a statistically significant difference between groups as determined by one-way ANOVA ($F(3,196) = 13.148, p = .000$). A Tukey post-hoc test revealed that there is statistically significant differences between the attitudes of Sanitary Staff & Doctors ($P = 0.000$) and Sanitary Staff and Laboratory Technicians ($P = 0.002$) and Nurses & Doctors ($P = 0.000$) and Nurses & Laboratory Technicians ($P = 0.003$) while there is no statistically significant differences between the attitudes of Sanitary Staff & Nurses ($P = 0.952$) and Doctors & Laboratory Technicians ($P = 0.765$) .

ANOVA

Summated.Attitude

	Sum of Squares	df	Mean Square	F	Sig.
Between Groups	359.655	3	119.885	13.148	.000
Within Groups	1787.125	196	9.118		
Total	2146.780	199			

Multiple Comparisons

Dependent Variable: Summated.Attitude

Tukey HSD

(I) Position	(J) Position	Mean Difference (I-J)	Std. Error	Sig.	95% Confidence Interval	
					Lower Bound	Upper Bound
Sanitary Staff	Lab Technician	-2.47500*	.67520	.002	-4.2246	-.7254
	Nurse	-.32500	.61637	.952	-1.9222	1.2722
	Doctor	-3.07500*	.61637	.000	-4.6722	-1.4778
Lab Technician	Sanitary Staff	2.47500*	.67520	.002	.7254	4.2246
	Nurse	2.15000*	.61637	.003	.5528	3.7472
	Doctor	-.60000	.61637	.765	-2.1972	.9972
Nurse	Sanitary Staff	.32500	.61637	.952	-1.2722	1.9222
	Lab Technician	-2.15000*	.61637	.003	-3.7472	-.5528
	Doctor	-2.75000*	.55130	.000	-4.1785	-1.3215
Doctor	Sanitary Staff	3.07500*	.61637	.000	1.4778	4.6722
	Lab Technician	.60000	.61637	.765	-.9972	2.1972
	Nurse	2.75000*	.55130	.000	1.3215	4.1785

*. The mean difference is significant at the 0.05 level.

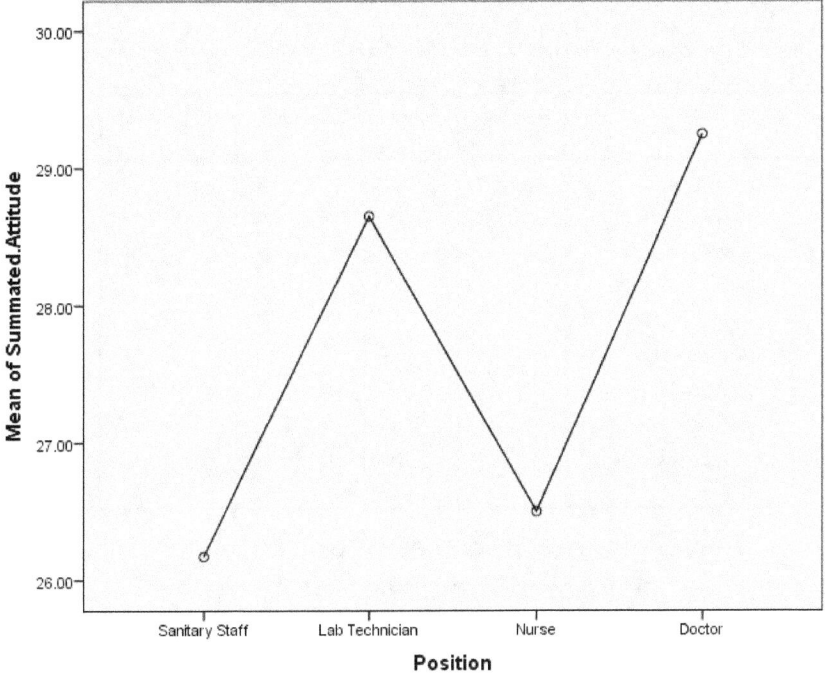

Practices:

Do you adopt any methods to protect yourself from the hazards of the waste during its management?

	Frequency	Percent	Valid Percent	Cumulative Percent
Nothing	19	9.5	9.5	9.5
Gloves	68	34.0	34.0	43.5
Masks	4	2.0	2.0	45.5
Gowns	1	.5	.5	46.0
Lab coats/boots	15	7.5	7.5	53.5
Gloves & Masks	31	15.5	15.5	69.0
Gloves & Gowns	3	1.5	1.5	70.5
Masks and Gown	1	.5	.5	71.0
Gloves Masks Gowns	58	29.0	29.0	100.0
Total	200	100.0	100.0	

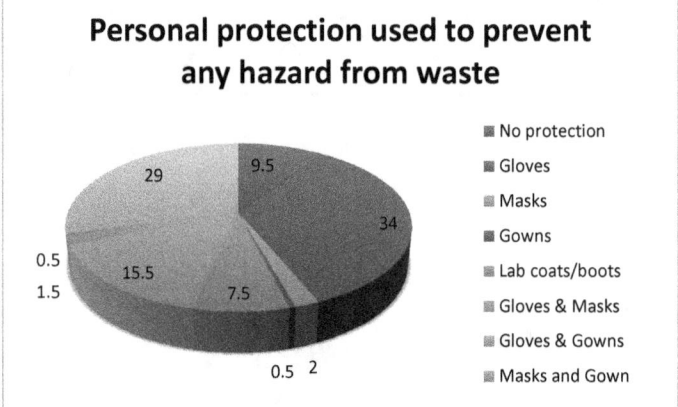

Personal protection used to prevent any hazard from waste

- No protection
- Gloves
- Masks
- Gowns
- Lab coats/boots
- Gloves & Masks
- Gloves & Gowns
- Masks and Gown

Are you (sanitary staff) satisfied with your working condition?

	Frequency	Percent	Valid Percent	Cumulative Percent
Yes	24	60.0	60.0	60.0
No	16	40.0	40.0	100.0
Total	40	100.0	100.0	

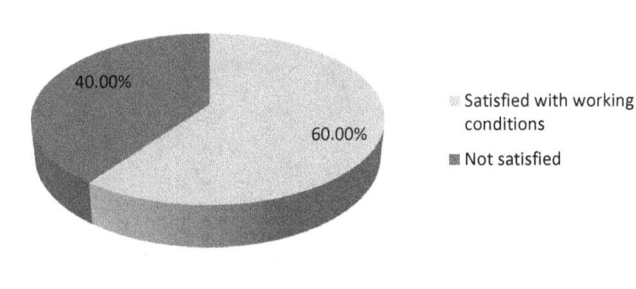

Waste managment staff satisfied with their working conditions

Reasons why the waste management staff not satisfied with their working condition

		Frequency	Percent	Valid Percent	Cumulative Percent
	Safety measures not sufficient	2	5.0	12.5	12.5
	Causing health risk	4	10.0	25.0	37.5
	Salary not sufficient	4	10.0	25.0	62.5
	Safety & health risk	2	5.0	12.5	75.0
	Safety & Salary	2	5.0	12.5	87.5
	Health risk and salary	2	5.0	12.5	100.0
	Total	16	40.0	100.0	
Missing	System	24	60.0		
Total		40	100.0		

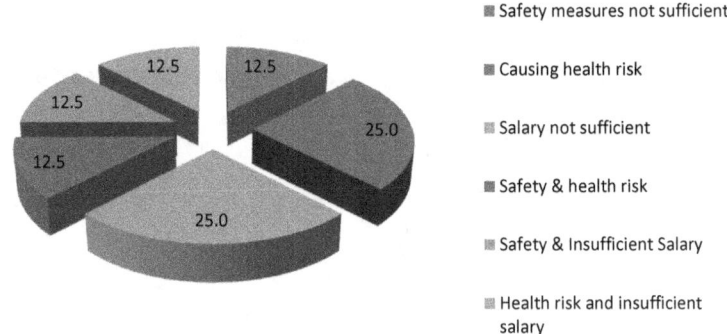

Reasons why the waste management staff not satisfied with their working condition

- Safety measures not sufficient
- Causing health risk
- Salary not sufficient
- Safety & health risk
- Safety & Insufficient Salary
- Health risk and insufficient salary

The practices exercised in the hospital for the segregation, collection,

transportation, storage, treatment and ultimate disposal were observed using an

"Observational Checklist" by a team of our students. It was found out that there is

no segregation of waste at the point of its origin at all. No different color-coded

bags etc., were used to segregate the different types of waste i.e. sharps, infectious,

pathological etc. The personal protection used by the doctors, nurses and

laboratory technicians to protect them from contamination or any hazards from this

waste are.

	Do you adopt any methods to protect yourself from the hazards of the waste during its management?								
	Nothing	Gloves	Masks	Gowns	Others	Gloves & Masks	Gloves & Gowns	Masks and Gown	Gloves Masks Gowns
Lab Technician	10.0%	40.0%	0.0%	0.0%	5.0%	15.0%	5.0%	0.0%	25.0%
Nurse	8.3%	5.0%	0.0%	0.0%	0.0%	26.7%	0.0%	1.7%	58.3%
Doctor	3.3%	45.0%	6.7%	1.7%	11.7%	11.7%	1.7%	0.0%	18.3%
Total	9.5%	34.0%	2.0%	.5%	7.5%	15.5%	1.5%	.5%	29.0%

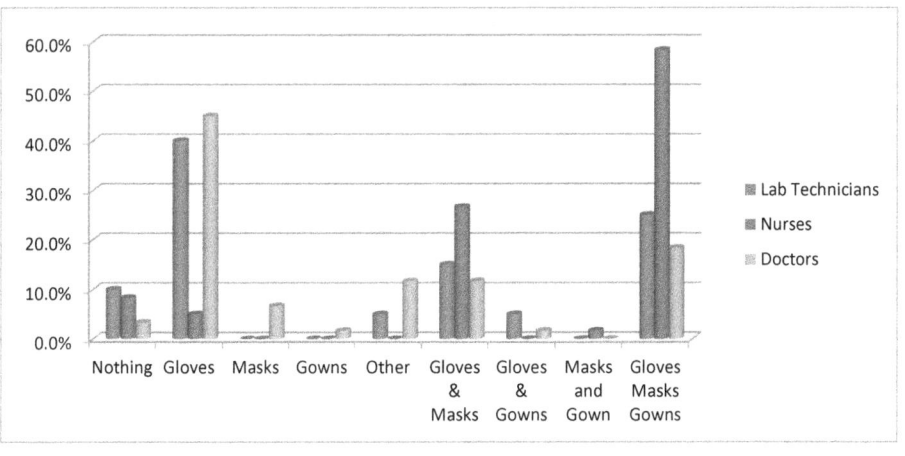

The waste was primarily collected in dustbins either internally lined by large plastic bags (shoppers) or without them. All the waste produced in wards, operation theatres went straight into these dustbins without any segregation process. The dustbins didn't have any "Biohazard Symbol" on them to indicate that it poses a potential threat to the living beings and should be handled with care and with self-protection.

The sanitary staff (sweepers) used to collect this waste from the wards, operation theatres and laboratories either in those shoppers which were placed in the bins or the dustbins as whole. The self-protection in sweepers were

	Do you adopt any methods to protect yourself from the hazards of the waste during its management?								
	No protection	Gloves	Masks	Gowns	Boots	Gloves & Masks	Gloves & Gowns	Masks and Gown	Gloves Masks Gowns
Sanitary Staff	20.0%	55.0%	0.0%	0.0%	15.0%	5.0%	0.0%	0.0%	5.0%

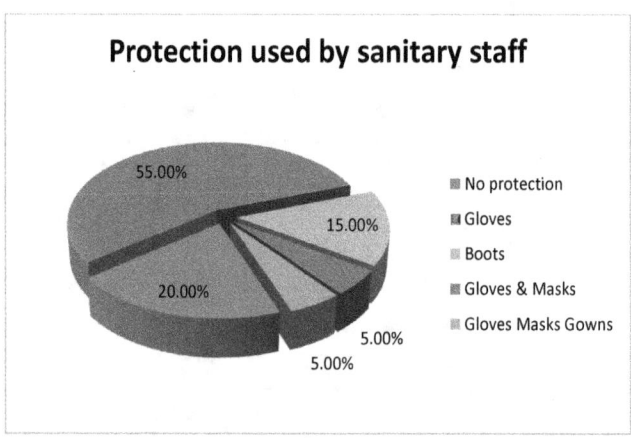

The waste from different wards was taken by a cart wheel or either in those shoppers to the waste storage site at the back of HMC which was an open dump. During the transportation of the waste no air tight or sealed packaging of the waste was made to prevent the contamination. Some of the waste fell down during its transportation. The waste was stored as open dump at the back of HMC near the incinerator. No measures were present to prevent the contamination of the nearby place from the waste or to prevent flying away of waste in the air with winds. From that dump paper and plastic is recollected which is then sold while the rest of waste is treated in the incinerator. An incinerator is present at the back of HMC for the treatment of waste.

DISCUSSION

The doctors and laboratory technicians had a better knowledge and awareness about biomedical waste handling and management as compared to the nurses and sanitary staff. The knowledge and awareness of the nurses was very low contrary to our expectations. Less than 10% of the nurses and sweepers knew what biomedical waste means. Only 46.7% of the doctors and 1.7% of the nurses knew the biohazard symbol. In another study at a tertiary care hospital of Rawalpindi 61% of doctors and 27% of nurses knew the biohazard symbol[8]. This shows that knowledge about biohazard symbol in our study is much less than that of the above mentioned study. Most of the staff was aware of the fact that improper management of medical waste poses a great level of risk and may cause different diseases like HBV, HCV and HIV & AIDS. Even about 90% of the sweepers knew that if this waste is not properly handled and disposed, it can cause diseases. Only 25% doctors, 10% laboratory technicians and only 1.7% of the nurses knew the use of color-coded bags for the collection of waste and the different color-coded bags and the type of waste disposed in each. In another study at a tertiary care hospital of Rawalpindi 86% doctors 86% nurses while 17% paramedics knew waste bin color-coding[8]. Almost half of the doctors, nurses, lab technicians and sweepers were unaware about their hospital waste management plan. Only 10% of the sweepers had received some training/attended workshops on waste and management and disposal. Similarly, most of the doctors, nurses and paramedics also haven't received any training or attended any seminars/workshops on waste management. These results are consistent with the finding of a study conducted at Allied Hospital Faisalabad for the evaluation of Infectious hospital waste during which It was revealed that hospital staff neither had knowledge regarding infectious hospital waste management nor were trained / properly equipped in the management of such specific waste[9]. Another study at the Combined Military Hospital, Rawalpindi, also showed that none of the sanitary workers had received any formal training in handling of hospital wastes[10].

The attitude of the doctors, nurses, lab technicians and sweepers about biomedical waste disposal and its significance was not up to the mark. The sanitary staff (sweepers) had the least summated attitude of 26.18 while 26.50, 28.65, 29.25 where the summated attitudes of nurses, laboratory technicians and doctors respectively. The maximum possible summated attitude was 35. The difference between 35 and doctors summated attitude is statistically significant ($P < 0.05$). A one way ANOVA test of these summated attitudes showed that the differences between attitude of different groups (Sanitary Staff, Laboratory Technicians, Nurses, Doctors) is statistically significant ($P < 0.05$). A Tukey post-hoc test revealed that there is statistically significant differences between the attitudes of Sanitary Staff & Doctors ($P = 0.000$) and Sanitary Staff and Laboratory Technicians ($P = 0.002$) and Nurses & Doctors ($P = 0.000$) and Nurses & Laboratory Technicians ($P = 0.003$) while there is no statistically significant differences between the attitudes of Sanitary Staff & Nurses ($P = 0.952$) and

Doctors & Laboratory Technicians ($P = 0.765$). The attitude differences can be partly due to the more education of the doctors than nurses and sweepers. But the summated attitude of nurses was much lower than expected and almost equalled to that of the sweepers. This may be partly because of the work burden on them and they considered it as an unnecessary burden. In another study at tertiary care hospital Kolkata, India, the summated attitudes of doctors and nurses were 25 and 21.5 respectively out of 30 (maximum possible summated attitude)[11]. There was no statistically significant difference between summated attitude of doctor and maximum possible summated attitude in that study, so their attitude can be rated as good[11]. A KAP study in urban area of Karachi evaluated the attitudes of sanitary workers, it was found that 38% sanitary had good (score of 9-15 out of maximum 15) and 62 % had poor (score of 1-8 out of maximum 15) attitude for the disposal of health-care facility waste[12].

Gloves were by far the most frequently used item used by the staff to protect them. The usage of other self-protection equipment was low. Forty Percent of the sweepers were not satisfied with their working conditions, mostly because they thought that there is a big risk to their own health and their salary is also insufficient. The waste handling and management methods were sub-standard. The findings of another study also suggested that there is no efficient system of disposal of solid hospital wastes in Pakistan[13]. No use of color-coding bags for collection of waste. The infectious waste was not segregated at the source. These results are consistent with the finding of a study conducted at Allied Hospital Faisalabad for the evaluation of Infectious hospital waste which also showed that there was no segregation of waste at the source of generation[9]. The waste is transported from wards in shoppers or open trolleys and then stored as an open dump near the incinerator from which the paper and plastic is separated and the rest are incinerated in the incinerator. The incinerator is treating their infectious as well as non-infectious waste together which is against the norm. The incinerator was polluting the air because of the toxic gases produced as a result of combustion of waste.

CONCLUSIONS

In the light of our study the following conclusions were made.

- The doctors and the laboratory technicians had better knowledge about biomedical waste, its management and handling than the nurses and the sanitary staff. Even more than half of the doctors didn't know about the biohazard symbol and the percentage was even extremely less in the nurses and sanitary staff. Almost all the staff had an adequate knowledge that improper management of this waste might cause different health problems.

Very little percentage of the staff has received any training/attended any workshop or seminar on biomedical waste disposal.

• Positive attitude towards biomedical waste disposal was highest in doctors followed by the laboratory technicians, nurses and was the least in sanitary staff. This clearly showed that those who have acquired higher education had a more positive attitude than the others.

• Gloves were widely used by the staff for self-protection. But still the sanitary staff was not in proper dress with proper mask, gloves, gown, boots to avoid the hazards of the waste. About half of the sanitary workers were not satisfied with their working conditions because according to them the salary was not sufficient and there was a risk to their health from this waste. No segregation at source and no use of color-coded bags. The waste is treated in an incinerator as a whole with no separate treatment of infectious and non-infectious components.

RECOMMENDATIONS

1. The staff should be educated about the concept of biomedical waste, and the precautionary measures they should take while its handling, management and disposal. The staff should also be educated about the different types of waste, the biohazard symbol, the use of color-coded bags for the collection of waste etc. The importance of proper management of biomedical waste should be emphasized and they should be made aware of the risks and

threats it poses to public health and environment if not properly managed and disposed.

2. Proper formal training should be given to the sanitary workers.

3. Seminars and workshops should be regularly conducted to emphasize the importance of biomedical waste disposal and to keep the procedures and techniques up to date.

4. A proper dress with masks, gloves, coat and boots etc. should be provided to the sanitary workers for their personal protection.

5. The salary of the sanitary workers should be reconsidered and increased.

6. The staff should be vaccinated, so that they remain protected even after an accidental mishap e.g. pricks from syringes.

7. The waste should be segregated at the source of generation.

8. Color-coded bags should be used for the collection of waste.

   • Yellow Bag: Infectious waste, bandages, gauze, cotton or any other objects in contact with body fluids, human body parts, placenta

   • Red: Plastic waste such as catheter, injections, syringes, tubings, IV bottles

   • Blue: All types of glass items and broken glass articles, out-dated and discarded medicines

   • Black: Needles without syringes, blades, sharps and all metal articles

9. The biohazard symbol should be pasted on containers which contain potential infectious substances.

10. The waste should be sealed and tightly packed. The waste should be transported with care.

11. It should be stored in a closed place for not more than 48 hours.

12. The infectious and non-infectious waste should be treated in the incinerated separately.

13. Measures should be taken to prevent the discharge of poisonous gases in the air.

14. The waste should be transported with care.

15. It should be stored in a closed room or place for not more than 48 hours.

16. Landfill disposal of the ashes and other non-infectious solid should be practiced.

Limitations

Annexures

Questionnaire Statement:

A knowledge, attitude & practices (KAP) survey of biomedical waste disposal in HMC

Personals

Name: _____

Age: _____

Sex: M ☐   F ☐

Ward: _____

Position

- Sanitary staff ☐
- Lab. Technician ☐
- Nurse ☐
- Doctor ☐

Educational Status:

- Primary ☐
- Matric ☐
- HSSC ☐
- Graduation ☐
- Post-Graduation ☐
- Others(Specify) _____

Knowledge

Q1. Have you heard about Biomedical Waste?

Yes ☐   No ☐

Q2. IF yes, what does it mean?

_____

_____

_____

Q3. Do you know about this symbol?

Yes ☐   No ☐

Q4. Are you aware that improper management of Biomedical Waste causes different health problems?

Yes ☐   No ☐

If yes which diseases

- HIV   ☐
- Hepatitis   ☐
- Any others, Specify

_____

Q5. Do you know the use of various types of color-coded bags for collection of Biomedical Waste?

Yes ☐   No ☐

Q6. If yes explain the different colours and the items disposed in them?

Yellow   _____

Red   _____

Blue   _____

Black   _____

Q7. Does your hospital have a Waste Management Plan?

Yes ☐   No ☐

Q8. Are there clearly defined procedures for collection and handling of wastes from specified units in the hospital?

Yes ☐   No ☐

Q9. Have you received any training/attended workshop on hospital waste management?

Yes ☐   No ☐

Q10. Are instructions/training given to newly hired waste management staff?(For sanitary staff only)

Yes ☐   No ☐

Attitude

1. Safe management of health care waste is an important issue
   - Strongly Disagree ☐
   - Disagree ☐
   - Undecided ☐
   - Agree ☐
   - Strongly Agree ☐
2. Management of healthcare waste is not the responsibility of doctors/nurses/paramedic staff
   - Strongly Disagree ☐
   - Disagree ☐
   - Undecided ☐
   - Agree ☐
   - Strongly Agree ☐
3. Waste management is possible even in overcrowded hospitals of Peshawar
   - Strongly Disagree ☐
   - Disagree ☐
   - Undecided ☐
   - Agree ☐
   - Strongly Agree ☐
4. Waste management efforts by hospitals need unnecessary expenditure
   - Strongly Disagree ☐
   - Disagree ☐
   - Undecided ☐
   - Agree ☐
   - Strongly Agree ☐

5. Safe management of waste is an extra burden on over-worked hospital staff
   - Strongly Disagree ☐
   - Disagree ☐
   - Undecided ☐
   - Agree ☐
   - Strongly Agree ☐

6. Waste management is possible even when patients are poor and illiterate
   - Strongly Disagree ☐
   - Disagree ☐
   - Undecided ☐
   - Agree ☐
   - Strongly Agree ☐

7. Proper segregation and then properly managed and disposed waste decrease the likelihood of the disease risk from the waste
   - Strongly Disagree ☐
   - Disagree ☐
   - Undecided ☐
   - Agree ☐
   - Strongly Agree ☐

Practice

1. Do you adopt any methods to protect yourself from the hazards of the waste during its management?
   - Gloves ☐
   - Masks ☐
   - Gowns ☐
   - Any other _____

2. Are you satisfied with your working condition?
   - Yes ☐
   - No ☐

   If no, why
   - Safety measures not sufficient ☐
   - Causing health risks ☐
   - Salary not sufficient ☐

Observation Checklist
Waste segregation, collection, storage, and handling

Handling of Segregated Waste	Sharps	Pathological Waste	Infectious waste	Radioactive waste	Chen wa:
Indicate by X the type of waste (in any) that is segregated from general waste stream.					
Where is the segregation taking place (i.e. operating room, laboratory, etc.)?					
What type of containers/bags (primary containment vessels) are used to segregate waste (bags, cardboard boxes, plastic containers, metal containers, etc.)? Describe accurately.					
What type of labelling, colour-coding (if any) is used for marking segregated waste? Describe					
1. Who handles (removes) the segregated waste (designation of the hospital staff member)? 2. Is the waste handler using any protective clothing (gloves, etc.) during waste handling? Yes/No.					
What type of containers (plastic bins, bags, cardboard boxes, trolleys, wheelbarrows, etc.) is used for collection and internal transport of the waste? Describe					
Where is the segregated waste stored while awaiting removal from the hospital or disposal? Describe.					
Describe briefly the final disposal of segregated waste (taken to municipal landfill, buried on hospital grounds, incinerated, open burned, etc.).					

References

1. Standard Operating Procedures SOPs for Hospital Waste Management Government of Pakistan, 1996

2. Chandra H. Hospital Waste And Its Management. In: *The World Environment Day. June 5,1999.*; July 1999

3. Mathur P, Patan S, Shobhawat S. Need of Biomedical Waste Management System in Hospitals - An Emerging issue - A Review. Curr World Environ 2012;7(1):117-124.

4. Hakeem Khattak F. Hospital Waste Management in Pakistan. *Pak J Med Res.* 2009; 48 (1)

5. Health-care waste management. *WHO Media Center.* 2011; Available from: http://www.who.int/mediacentre/factsheets/fs281/en/ [Accessed 20 Sep 2013].

6. *Dr. Ijaz Ahmad, Review Of Current Waste Management Strategies.* At Public And Private Sector Hospitals Of Islamabad

7. Ministry of Environment, Government of Pakistan *Hospital Waste Management Rules, 2005.* [Press release] 3rd August, 2005 2005. Ministry of Environment, Government of Pakistan *Hospital Waste Management Rules, 2005.* [Press release] 3rd August, 2005

8. Kumar R, Ali Gorar Z, Khan Z, Ali Z. ASSESSMENT OF HEALTH CARE WASTE MANAGEMENT PRACTICES AND KNOWLEDGE AMONG HEALTH CARE WORKERS WORKING AT TERTIARY CARE SETTING OF PAKISTAN. *Journal of Health Research.* 2013; 27,2013 (4): 5.

9. Johri AE, Goraya JA, Maqbool R. Evaluation of infectious Hospital Waste Management at the Allied Hospital Faisalabad. Pak J Health. 1998; 35: 106-9.

10. Muhammed Ashraf Chaudry, Azhar Hayat, Shaukat Mahmood Qureshi, Syed Abdul Ahad Najimi. Health hazard of hospital waste to sanitary workers at Combined Military Hospital, Rawalpindi.Pak Armed Forces Med J Dec 2004; 54: 253-8.

11. Chattopadhyay D, Bisoi S, Biswas B, Chattopadhyay S. Study of attitude regarding health care waste management among health care providers of a tertiary care hospital in Kolkata. Indian J Public Health 2010;54:104-5

12. Habibullah S, Afsar S. Waste Disposal of Government Health-Care Facilities in Urban Area of Karachi - A KAP Survey. *Pak J Med Res.* 2007; 46 (1)

13. Khan MR, Fareedi F, Rashid B. Techno-economic disposal of hospital wastes in Pakistan. Pak J Med Res 2006; 45: 41-5

14. Annual Report 2009, Hayatabad Medical Complex, Peshawar.

www.ingramcontent.com/pod-product-compliance
Lightning Source LLC
Chambersburg PA
CBHW071825200526
45169CB00018B/1026